MSM

A Beginner's Quick Start Guide and Overview of Its Use Cases, with a Potential 3-Step Plan on Getting Started copyright © 2023 Tyler Spellmann

All rights reserved No part of this book may be reproduced, or stored in a retrieval system, or transmitted in any form or by any means, electronic, mechanical, photocopying, recording, or otherwise, without express written permission of the publisher.

Disclaimer

By reading this disclaimer, you are accepting the terms of the disclaimer in full. If you disagree with this disclaimer, please do not read the guide.

All of the content within this guide is provided for informational and educational purposes only, and should not be accepted as independent medical or other professional advice. The author is not a doctor, physician, nurse, mental health provider, or registered nutritionist/dietician. Therefore, using and reading this guide does not establish any form of a physician-patient relationship.

Always consult with a physician or another qualified health provider with any issues or questions you might have regarding any sort of medical condition. Do not ever disregard any qualified professional medical advice or delay seeking that advice because of anything you have read in this guide. The information in this guide is not intended to be any sort of medical advice and should not be used in lieu of any medical advice by a licensed and qualified medical professional.

The information in this guide has been compiled from a variety of known sources. However, the author cannot attest to or guarantee the accuracy of each source and thus should not be held liable for any errors or omissions.

You acknowledge that the publisher of this guide will not be held liable for any loss or damage of any kind incurred as a result of this guide or the reliance on any information provided within this guide. You acknowledge and agree that you assume all risk and responsibility for any action you undertake in response to the information in this guide.

Using this guide does not guarantee any particular result (e.g., weight loss or a cure). By reading this guide, you acknowledge that there are no guarantees to any specific outcome or results you can expect.

All product names, diet plans, or names used in this guide are for identification purposes only and are the property of their respective owners. The use of these names does not imply endorsement. All other trademarks cited herein are the property of their respective owners.

Where applicable, this guide is not intended to be a substitute for the original work of this diet plan and is, at most, a supplement to the original work for this diet plan and never a direct substitute. This guide is a personal expression of the facts of that diet plan.

Where applicable, persons shown in the cover images are stock photography models and the publisher has obtained the rights to use the images through license agreements with third-party stock image companies.

Table of Contents

Introduction — 6
What Is Methylsulphonylmethane (MSM)? — 8
   How Does It Work? — 9
   Benefits of Methylsulfonylmethane (MSM) — 10
   Various Forms of Methylsulfonylmethane (MSM) — 13
Use Cases of Methylsulphonylmethane (MSM) — 18
   Arthritis and joint pain — 18
   Allergies and respiratory issues — 19
   Skin conditions — 19
   Digestive issues — 20
   Athletic performance — 20
Pros and Cons of MSM — 22
   Advantages of Methylsulfonylmethane — 22
   Disadvantages of Methylsulphonylmethane (MSM) — 26
Recommended Dosage and Usage — 28
   Potential Side Effects of Methylsulfonylmethane (MSM) — 29
3-Step Plan to Getting Started with Methylsulfonylmethane (MSM) — 32
   Step 1: Consult with a healthcare professional — 32
   Step 2: Choose a high-quality MSM supplement — 33
   Step 3: Start with a low dose and gradually increase — 33
Safety Precautions and Considerations — 35
   Who Can Take Methylsulfonylmethane (MSM) — 39
Food Sources of Methylsulfonylmethane (MSM) — 42
   How diet can play a role in getting enough Methylsulfonylmethane (MSM) — 44
Conclusion — 46
FAQ — 49
References and Helpful Links — 52

Introduction

Are you struggling with inflammation, joint pain, or digestive issues? If so, you're not alone. These health issues affect millions of people worldwide and can significantly impact their quality of life. However, there may be a natural solution that can help alleviate these symptoms - MSM.

MSM is a naturally occurring compound found in fruits, vegetables, grains, and even milk. It is known for its anti-inflammatory properties, making it an excellent choice for those seeking relief from joint pain and other inflammatory conditions. Additionally, MSM has been shown to aid in digestion by reducing bloating, gas, and other digestive discomforts.

The benefits of MSM on overall health and wellness are hard to ignore. Not only does it have anti-inflammatory properties, but it also aids in digestion, making it an excellent choice for those looking to improve their gut health. Furthermore, MSM can help improve skin health and reduce the signs of aging.

In this guide, we will talk about the following in full detail:

- What is Methylsulphonylmethane (MSM)?
- How does Methylsulphonylmethane (MSM) Work?
- Various Forms Of Methylsulphonylmethane (MSM)
- Benefits, Advantages, and Disadvantages Of Methylsulphonylmethane (MSM)
- Use Cases
- Recommended Dosage and Usage
- Potential Side Effects of Methylsulphonylmethane (MSM)
- 3-Step Plan to Get Started With Methylsulphonylmethane (MSM)
- Safety Precautions and Considerations
- Food Sources of Methylsulphonylmethane (MSM)
- How diet can play a role in getting enough Methylsulfonylmethane (MSM)

Keep reading to discover the science behind MSM and learn more about its potential health benefits. By the end of this guide, you will have a better understanding of how MSM works and whether or not it could be a helpful supplement for your overall health and wellness goals. So, let's dive in!

What Is Methylsulphonylmethane (MSM)?

Methylsulfonylmethane (MSM) is a naturally occurring organic compound that contains Sulfur. Sulfur is an essential nutrient that our bodies need for various functions, such as building healthy cells, producing collagen, and maintaining joint health. MSM is derived from dimethyl sulfoxide (DMSO), which was first synthesized in 1866.

Methylsulfonylmethane (MSM) was discovered in the early 1980s when researchers were studying DMSO when they realized that MSM was a metabolite of the original compound and shared similar anti-inflammatory properties.

Its popularity has grown in recent years due to its potential benefits for pain relief, joint health, and skincare. It is available in various forms such as capsules, tablets, powders, creams, and gels, and is commonly used by people looking for a natural approach to health and wellness.

How Does It Work?

Methylsulfonylmethane, also known as MSM, is a chemical that occurs naturally and is composed of sulfur. It is believed that it works in the body by supplying the sulfur that is necessary for the production of other vital chemicals such as glutathione, which is a potent antioxidant that assists in the detoxification of the body and helps minimize oxidative stress.

MSM is also known to have anti-inflammatory effects, which can help reduce inflammation, swelling, and discomfort in the body. These benefits can be obtained with regular use of MSM.

When taken orally, MSM is absorbed into the bloodstream and circulated throughout the body, where it is able to give the sulfur that is required to support a variety of processes throughout the body. In particular, it has been demonstrated that MSM can improve joint health by lowering inflammation and encouraging the creation of collagen.

Collagen is a protein that can be found in cartilage as well as other connective tissues. Because of this, it can be used as an effective natural cure for the pain and stiffness in the joints that are associated with illnesses such as osteoarthritis and rheumatoid arthritis.

MSM is used directly on the skin in the form of creams and lotions in order to promote skin health and reduce the appearance of signs of aging. It is thought to operate by boosting the body's natural production of collagen and lowering inflammatory levels in the skin.

MSM is also applied directly to the scalp in the form of hair care products in order to promote healthier hair, faster hair growth, and less hair loss. It is said to function by increasing the amount of blood that flows to the scalp and providing the hair follicles with the critical nutrients they need.

In general, the precise process of how MSM works in the body is not completely understood; but, due to its various health benefits, it has become a popular natural supplement for a wide range of health conditions.

Benefits of Methylsulfonylmethane (MSM)

Studies have shown that MSM may be effective in treating several health issues, from joint pain and inflammation to allergies. Here are some of the potential benefits of MSM:

Reduces inflammation

It has been established that MSM possesses anti-inflammatory qualities, which make it capable of assisting in the reduction of inflammation throughout the body and the alleviation of joint pain. Inflammation is a natural response that occurs when the body is wounded or under stress; however, persistent inflammation can contribute to a variety of health concerns.

Inflammation is a natural response that occurs when the body is harmed or under stress. Due to the fact that it has anti-inflammatory characteristics, MSM could be a beneficial supplement for people who suffer from illnesses like arthritis or fibromyalgia, both of which are characterized by chronic inflammation.

Improves skin health

It has been shown that MSM can provide the skin with a number of different benefits. It does this by lowering inflammation and boosting the production of collagen, both of which contribute to an overall improvement in the skin's appearance and texture.

This can help lessen the indications of aging. Due to the anti-inflammatory characteristics that MSM possesses, it may also be beneficial for people who suffer from skin disorders such as eczema, psoriasis, or rosacea.

Boosts immune system

Methylsulfonylmethane has been demonstrated to possess immune-enhancing qualities, which positions it as a possible natural remedy for enhancing general health and wellness. MSM contains the necessary mineral sulfur, which stimulates the production of glutathione within the body.

Glutathione is a potent antioxidant that plays an important part in the immune system. It is well known that glutathione has the ability to scavenge free radicals as well as assist the functioning of the immune system. MSM also possesses anti-inflammatory qualities, which make it an effective tool for lowering oxidative stress, a factor that has been associated with impaired immunological function.

Relieves allergies

MSM is a powerful natural remedy that can help with allergy symptoms. According to some studies, it has the ability to inhibit the release of histamine, which is the chemical that sets off allergic reactions. As a result, allergy symptoms including sneezing, watery eyes, and difficulty breathing are alleviated.

Additionally, it can reduce inflammation in the sinuses and airways, making it easier to breathe as a result. It has also been demonstrated that MSM can strengthen the immune system, which can help lower the intensity of the symptoms associated with allergic reactions. Those who suffer from allergies and use MSM on a daily basis may discover that they are able to find some relief without having to turn to more powerful drugs.

Supports healthy bones and joints

MSM is a valuable supplement for persons who suffer from osteoporosis or arthritis since it can help increase joint flexibility and reduce inflammation in the joints. MSM may also assist in maintaining bone health by enhancing calcium absorption and lowering calcium excretion, both of which can help to avoid the gradual loss of bone density that comes with aging.

In addition, the anti-inflammatory characteristics of MSM can assist in the alleviation of joint discomfort and stiffness, making it simpler to lead an active lifestyle.

Overall, MSM has a wide range of potential health benefits and may be a useful supplement for those looking to improve their overall health and well-being. However, as with any supplement, it's important to choose a reputable brand, follow the recommended dosage, and consult with a healthcare provider before starting any new supplement regimen.

Various Forms of Methylsulfonylmethane (MSM)

Methylsulfonylmethane (MSM) is available in a variety of forms, including;

Capsules and Tablets

Consuming Methylsulfonylmethane in the form of MSM capsules or tablets is a method that is both practical and effective. MSM capsules normally come in quantities ranging from 500 mg to 1500 mg, although the amount of MSM included in a single tablet dosing can range anywhere from 1000 mg to 5000 mg. People who are constantly on the move but still need to achieve their daily MSM consumption needs will find these forms to be very user-friendly and convenient.

In addition, MSM capsules are frequently utilized for the management of joint discomfort and inflammation, whereas MSM tablets are mostly utilized for the enhancement of healthy hair, skin, and nails. In spite of the differences in their applications, both types of methylsulfonylmethane are widely used because of how efficient and beneficial they are.

Powder

MSM powder is another form of compound that can be easily consumed by mixing it with liquids such as smoothies, juices, and other drinks. In addition to this, it can also be combined with topical products such as lotions and creams in order to improve the efficacy of those products for maintaining healthy skin. The amount of MSM powder contained in a single serving might range anywhere from 500 mg to 5000 mg, depending on the product that was purchased.

Topical Cream

MSM topical creams are an efficient method for increasing the amount of MSM present in the body. Because the cream is applied directly to the skin, absorption can be facilitated in a timely and directed manner. MSM is well-known for the anti-inflammatory effects that it possesses; hence, it is a common treatment option for those who are afflicted with ailments such as arthritis, tendonitis, and muscle discomfort.

Additionally, MSM creams frequently contain natural substances such as aloe vera and coconut oil, both of which can further boost the health of the skin and the skin's ability to retain moisture. MSM topical creams are available in a range of concentrations to cater to the specific requirements of each individual, and using these creams is a practical and uncomplicated approach to including MSM in one's regular skincare routine.

Liquid

Methylsulfonylmethane (MSM) is available in a variety of forms, one of which is the liquid MSM. MSM is dissolved in water throughout the manufacturing process, which results in a highly concentrated solution that is simple to take orally. Those people who have trouble swallowing tablets or capsules are perfect candidates for the liquid version, which can also be mixed into other liquids such as water, juice, or smoothies to make them easier to consume.

In addition to this, the liquid form of MSM is readily absorbed by the body and is an excellent supply of sulfur, which is necessary for maintaining healthy hair, skin, and nails. When selecting an MSM liquid, it is crucial to look for solutions that are of high quality and free from impurities; therefore, it is important to always read the label and select a brand that has a good reputation.

Crystals

Consuming or using Methylsulfonylmethane (MSM) in the form of MSM crystals is a method that is diverse as well as convenient. This particular kind of MSM can be dissolved in water and taken orally, or it can be applied topically and used as a supplement.

MSM crystals, as opposed to pills or capsules, offer a one-of-a-kind alternative to consumers who would rather take their MSM in a different form. In addition, MSM crystals are well-known for their lack of impurities and high levels of potency, which makes them an excellent option for people who are looking for high-quality MSM supplements.

Gel

Because of its potential to alleviate pain and because of its anti-inflammatory actions, MSM gel is a popular topical therapy. Methylsulfonylmethane (MSM), a naturally occurring chemical that may be found in both plants and animals, is included in the formulation of the gel. It is thought that MSM works by lowering levels of oxidative stress and inflammation in the body, both of which are thought to play a big part in how one experiences pain.

MSM gel has the ability to be applied directly to the skin, allowing it to have a calming impact on the body while also being utilized to target specific parts of the body. Although additional research is required to verify its efficacy, numerous users of MSM gel have reported experiencing great pain alleviation after using the product.

It's important to note that the recommended dosage and effectiveness of MSM may vary depending on the specific form of MSM you are using. Always follow the recommended dosages on the product label or as directed by your healthcare provider.

Use Cases of Methylsulphonylmethane (MSM)

In this chapter, we will explore the use cases of MSM and its associated benefits. Whether you're looking to boost your immune system or reduce chronic pain, MSM may be a natural and safe solution for your health needs.

Arthritis and joint pain

Because of its anti-inflammatory effects, MSM can be an effective dietary supplement for people who suffer from arthritis or joint discomfort. MSM is able to ease pain and stiffness in the joints, enhance mobility, and prevent further damage to the joints by lowering the level of inflammation in the joints.

According to the findings of several studies, methylsulfonylmethane (MSM) may be especially helpful for those who suffer from osteoarthritis, a typical form of arthritis that develops as the cartilage that lines the joints wears away over time. Even though additional research is required to completely understand the benefits of MSM for arthritis and joint pain, a significant number of people have experienced beneficial results from using MSM as a supplement.

Allergies and respiratory issues

Because of its capacity to reduce inflammation and enhance respiratory function, MSM may be beneficial for people who suffer from allergies or respiratory conditions like asthma or sinusitis. MSM can help decrease allergy symptoms such as sneezing and coughing by lowering inflammation in the respiratory system.

This can also help reduce congestion, which can make it easier to breathe, and lessen breathing difficulties. According to the findings of a few studies, MSM may also be beneficial for people who suffer from seasonal allergies, helping to improve their general quality of life throughout allergy season.

Skin conditions

Because of its antioxidant and anti-inflammatory characteristics, MSM may be helpful for those whose skin disorders include eczema, psoriasis, or rosacea. MSM can help improve overall skin health and minimize symptoms such as redness, flakiness, and itching by lowering inflammation and boosting the formation of collagen.

MSM can also help improve overall skin health. In addition, there is some evidence that MSM can help boost the skin's natural defenses against the toxins and damage caused by the environment, which can contribute to the skin appearing healthy and youthful.

Digestive issues

People who suffer from digestive disorders including irritable bowel syndrome (IBS) or leaky gut syndrome may find that taking MSM supplements is beneficial. MSM can help ease symptoms such as bloating, gas, cramps, and diarrhea by lowering inflammation in the gut. These symptoms might be caused by irritable bowel syndrome (IBS).

Additionally, there is some evidence to suggest that MSM can assist increase the growth of healthy gut bacteria and improve nutrient absorption, both of which are beneficial to the digestive system as a whole. Even though additional research is necessary to completely understand the benefits of MSM for digestive disorders, a lot of people have discovered that taking MSM in supplement form helps them feel better.

Athletic performance

Athletes and those who exercise frequently may benefit from taking MSM, as it has been found to offer potential health advantages in this population. MSM can aid increase recovery times and promote overall sports performance by lowering the amount of muscle damage and pain that is experienced.

In addition, there is some evidence that MSM can assist increase joint flexibility, making it simpler to move around and lowering the risk of injury while exercising. According to the findings of several studies, MSM may also be useful in lowering oxidative stress, which is a typical issue faced by athletes and is brought on by strenuous physical exercise.

Although additional research is required to completely understand the effects of MSM on athletic performance, numerous athletes have reported favorable outcomes after taking MSM as a dietary supplement.

These are only a handful of the many possible applications for MSM that could be developed. It is essential to have a conversation with your healthcare professional before beginning to take an MSM supplement in order to assess whether or not the supplement is appropriate for you and your specific health requirements.

Pros and Cons of MSM

In this section, we will discuss the advantages and disadvantages of methylsulfonylmethane (MSM).

Advantages of Methylsulfonylmethane

MSM, or Methylsulfonylmethane, has several advantages that make it an appealing supplement for those looking to improve their overall health and well-being. Some of the advantages of MSM include:

Natural

Methylsulphonylmethane, also known as MSM, is a totally natural substance that may be found in a wide variety of foods, such as cereals, fruits, and vegetables. In addition, it is offered in the form of dietary supplements, which are sourced from natural sources such as pine trees.

MSM is a natural compound that happens in nature, in contrast to synthetic compounds or drugs. Because of this, it may be intriguing to those who are looking for natural solutions to support their health because it occurs naturally.

Safe

When taken as directed, methylsulphonylmethane, also known as MSM, is not thought to pose a health risk to most people. Even when administered in high dosages, it hasn't been linked to any significant adverse effects and has a low risk of causing harm to the body.

Because of this, individuals can use MSM to support their health without worrying about the potential risks that are connected with using other supplements or pharmaceuticals. This makes it possible for individuals to use MSM with confidence.

Easy-to-use

MSM supplements are readily available in powder or capsule form, and it is simple to work them into one's routine. They normally consist solely of methylsulfonylmethane (MSM) and do not include any other components or fillers, which makes them a practical and uncomplicated choice of supplement.

Individuals can effortlessly incorporate MSM into their morning smoothie, incorporate it into their preferred beverage, or take it in tablet form along with their other regular vitamins and supplements.

Versatile

MSM, or methylsulphonylmethane, is a supplement that has several applications and can be used to treat a wide range of health conditions. Because of its anti-inflammatory and antioxidant characteristics, it is useful for a number of different aspects of health, including the health of the skin, the digestive tract, the respiratory system, and the joints.

Individuals are able to streamline their supplement routine and save money on the purchase of several supplements as a result of MSM's ability to support multiple aspects of their health.

Non-Addictive

The fact that methylsulphonylmethane (MSM) does not have an addictive property is a huge benefit when compared to the many other chemicals that have the potential to produce dependence and withdrawal symptoms. MSM can be used to maintain one's health without the user having to worry about getting dependent on the supplement in any way.

In addition, research has shown that taking MSM over a longer period of time can deliver several health benefits without the negative effects that are typically linked with substance dependence. Because it does not cause addiction, MSM is an approach that can help people keep up a healthy lifestyle in a way that is both sustainable and risk-free.

Affordable

MSM is well-known for its reasonable price, which makes it a well-liked choice among individuals who wish to improve their health without spending an excessive amount of money. MSM is typically sold at a price that is quite a bit lower than that of other supplements, which places it within the reach of a substantially larger population.

This indicates that even individuals who may have financial constraints can still make their health a priority by adding MSM into their daily routines. Additionally, due to the fact that it is very inexpensive, users are able to acquire MSM in greater quantities, thereby ensuring a consistent supply for continued use.

In the end, the fact that MSM is available at a price that is affordable is a big advantage that makes it a decision that is both accessible and practical for people who are looking to improve their general well-being.

Overall, MSM has several advantages that make it a promising supplement for those looking to improve their health and well-being naturally. However, as with any supplement, it's important to choose a reputable brand, follow the recommended dosage, and consult with a healthcare provider before starting any new supplement regimen.

Disadvantages of Methylsulphonylmethane (MSM)

Despite its potential benefits, there are a few disadvantages to using MSM as a supplement. These include:

Not suitable for everyone

Even while MSM is usually regarded to be harmless, some people may be allergic to it, and others may find that taking it causes stomach distress. It is essential to see a medical professional before beginning to take MSM supplements, particularly if you have a family history of allergic reactions or digestive problems.

On the basis of your specific health requirements and past medical history, your physician will be able to assist you in determining whether or not MSM is risk-free and appropriate for you to use.

May interact with certain medications

MSM has the potential to have an adverse effect when combined with a number of medications, including insulin and blood thinners. This is due to the fact that MSM has the tendency to amplify the effects of the drugs being taken. Because of this, it is essential to confer with a qualified medical expert prior to beginning treatment with MSM.

In addition, it is crucial that you inform your doctor about any drugs that you are currently taking, as they will be able to advise you on any necessary adjustments to the dosage in order to reduce the likelihood of adverse effects.

If you do not follow these instructions, you run the risk of experiencing more severe adverse effects or even consequences that could be fatal. Because of this, it is extremely important to use extreme caution when combining MSM consumption with the use of other drugs.

Limited research

In spite of the fact that there is some evidence to show that MSM may have a number of positive effects on one's health, additional research is required to completely understand both the possible advantages and risks associated with its use.

MSM has been the subject of a few studies; however, additional, more in-depth research is required to ascertain both its short-term and long-term effects, as well as how it interacts with other supplements and drugs. As a result, it is essential to approach MSM with caution and consult a physician before beginning to take it in order to confirm that it is both safe and suitable for your needs.

Despite its potential benefits, there are a few disadvantages to using MSM as a supplement. It's important to be aware of these before starting an MSM regimen and to consult with your healthcare provider if you have any questions or concerns.

Recommended Dosage and Usage

Although methylsulfonylmethane (MSM) is regularly used as a natural supplement, there is no known ideal dosage for any particular ailment. This is despite the fact that MSM is commonly used to treat symptoms of osteoarthritis and other inflammatory illnesses.

For osteoarthritis, people have tried taking anywhere from 500 milligrams of MSM twice daily to 3 grams once daily, but there is no standardized amount that has been scientifically confirmed to be beneficial. People have tried using MSM for osteoarthritis. In addition, the quality of MSM supplements, as well as the active components that they include, can fluctuate substantially from one manufacturer to the next, which makes it challenging to formulate a dosage schedule that is reliable.

Before beginning a regimen of MSM, it is vital to speak with a healthcare practitioner, just as it is with any other supplement, in order to identify the appropriate dosage and usage based on the individual's specific needs and current state of health.

Potential Side Effects of Methylsulfonylmethane (MSM)

While MSM is generally considered safe at recommended doses, there are some potential side effects and interactions to be aware of. Here are a few things to keep in mind:

Mild side effects

MSM, or methylsulphonylmethane, is a dietary supplement that has been shown to have a number of positive impacts on one's health, despite the possibility that it could also have some negative consequences. MSM is known to cause a number of unpleasant side effects, the most prevalent of which is diarrhea, which may also be accompanied by nausea and bloating.

Taking excessive doses of the supplement or using it for a lengthy period of time both increase the likelihood that this will occur. As a side effect of using MSM, some consumers have reported experiencing headaches. Before taking any kind of supplement, including MSM, it is essential to check with a medical professional to make sure that you won't be putting your health in danger.

Interactions with blood thinners

The influence that methylsulphonylmethane (MSM) has on blood-thinning drugs like warfarin is one of the more severe adverse effects of this substance. It has been discovered that

MSM can boost the efficiency of blood thinners, which in turn can lead to an increased risk of bleeding.

Because of this, those who use blood thinners should discuss the use of MSM with their physician before beginning treatment, as doing so may have adverse effects.

Interactions with diabetes medications

Methylsulphonylmethane, also known as MSM, has been shown to drop blood sugar levels in some people who take it; because of this, using it with diabetes treatment could be dangerous. Before using MSM, diabetics who are currently taking medication for their condition ought to keep a close eye on their blood sugar levels and discuss the matter with their primary care physician.

It's possible that taking the supplement will lower your blood sugar, which could put you at risk for hypoglycemia or other issues. In light of this risk, it is absolutely necessary to consult a physician before combining MSM consumption with diabetes treatment in any way.

Allergic reactions

It is known that methylsulphonylmethane, more commonly known as MSM, can trigger allergic reactions in certain people, particularly those who already have an allergy to sulfa-containing medications. Allergic reactions like these can cause a wide range of symptoms, including hives, itching, swelling, and difficulty breathing.

It is essential to keep in mind that even though they are uncommon, serious allergic reactions might take place and might call for rapid medical assistance. It is recommended that people who are sensitive to sulfa medicines or have a sensitivity to MSM avoid using it and instead see a healthcare expert prior to taking any supplements that include MSM.

It's always a good idea to consult with a healthcare professional before starting any new supplement regimen, especially if you have any underlying health conditions or are taking medications. They can help you determine if MSM is safe and appropriate for you to take, and guide dosage and potential interactions.

3-Step Plan to Getting Started with Methylsulfonylmethane (MSM)

If you're interested in incorporating MSM into your daily routine, here is a simple three-step guide to help you get started:

Step 1: Consult with a healthcare professional

Before starting an MSM regimen, it's essential to consult with a healthcare professional. MSM supplements can interact with certain medications, and it's crucial to ensure that they will not cause any adverse effects. Additionally, a healthcare professional can help determine the optimal dosage and usage based on individual needs and health status.

During your consultation, be sure to discuss any pre-existing medical conditions or medications you are currently taking. Your healthcare professional can help determine if MSM is right for you and provide guidance on how to incorporate it into your daily routine.

Step 2: Choose a high-quality MSM supplement

Once you have consulted with a healthcare professional, it's time to choose a high-quality MSM supplement. MSM supplements are available in various forms, including capsules, powders, and creams.

When choosing an MSM supplement, it's essential to look for a reputable brand that uses high-quality ingredients and has been independently tested for purity and potency. Additionally, look for a supplement that contains pure MSM without any fillers or additives.

Capsules and powders are the most common forms of MSM supplements. Capsules are convenient and easy to take, while powders can be easily added to smoothies or other beverages. MSM creams are also available for topical application to aid in skin health and reduce inflammation.

It's important to note that MSM supplements are not regulated by the FDA, and quality can vary widely between different manufacturers. Be sure to do your research and choose a reputable brand.

Step 3: Start with a low dose and gradually increase

Due to the lack of established optimal dosages for MSM, it's important to start with a low dose and gradually increase it to determine the optimal dosage for your individual needs. Your healthcare professional can help determine an appropriate starting dose based on your health status and any pre-existing conditions.

When incorporating MSM into your daily routine, start with the lowest recommended dose and gradually increase over time. This allows your body to adjust to the supplement and helps you determine the optimal dosage that works best for you.

It's important to note that MSM supplements may take several weeks or even months to see results. Be patient and consistent with your MSM regimen to reap its potential benefits.

If you experience any adverse effects, such as gastrointestinal discomfort or allergic reactions, discontinue use and consult with a healthcare professional.

Incorporating Methylsulfonylmethane (MSM) into your daily routine can potentially improve your overall health and wellness. However, it's essential to consult with a healthcare professional, choose a high-quality MSM supplement, start with a low dose, and gradually increase to determine the optimal dosage for your individual needs. Taking these steps can help ensure safety and efficacy and potentially improve your quality of life.

Safety Precautions and Considerations

Methylsulfonylmethane (MSM) is generally safe at recommended doses for short-term use. However, there are a few important safety precautions and considerations to be aware of:

Consult with a healthcare provider

When taking Methylsulfonylmethane (MSM), it is important to exercise caution if you are taking certain medications, such as chemotherapeutic therapies or immunosuppressants, as they may interact with MSM. To ensure your safety, it is recommended that you consult with your primary care physician before starting MSM supplementation.

It is important to note that MSM is generally considered safe for most individuals, but it is best to err on the side of caution and speak with a healthcare professional if you are taking any medications. Doing so can help you avoid any potential adverse reactions or side effects.

Follow recommended dosages

It is important to exercise caution and adhere to the recommended dosages when taking Methylsulfonylmethane (MSM). Though MSM is generally safe, exceeding the suggested quantities can result in unpleasant side effects like diarrhea and stomach distress. One should always follow the instructions provided on the product label or as directed by a healthcare provider to avoid any adverse reactions.

Avoid use during pregnancy and breastfeeding

Methylsulfonylmethane (MSM) is not recommended for pregnant and breastfeeding women due to insufficient evidence regarding its safety during these periods. It is important for women to avoid taking MSM supplements to avoid any potential risks that could harm them or their babies.

Instead, they should consult with their healthcare provider to determine safer options or to discuss the potential benefits and drawbacks of using MSM during pregnancy and breastfeeding. It is always better to err on the side of caution when it comes to the health and well-being of mothers and their babies.

Be cautious with kidney problems

Individuals who are considering taking Methylsulfonylmethane (MSM) should take note that the compound is primarily expelled from the body through the kidneys. Therefore, those who have preexisting kidney problems or issues should exercise caution before taking MSM.

Prior consultation with their primary care physician is crucial in avoiding any potential adverse effects that may arise from taking MSM. This is because MSM may further damage already compromised kidneys, leading to further complications and detrimental effects on their overall health.

Be aware of potential side effects

When taking Methylsulfonylmethane (MSM), it's crucial to be mindful of potential side effects and adverse reactions. While MSM is generally deemed safe, there is a possibility of gastrointestinal issues, headaches, or lethargy. These symptoms should not be ignored, and if experienced, the individual should cease usage and consult a healthcare professional.

Avoid use with certain medications

When taking Methylsulfonylmethane (MSM), it is important to exercise caution and avoid its use with certain medications. Certain chemotherapeutic therapies and immunosuppressants may interact with MSM and cause negative side effects.

Individuals who are taking medication should consult with their primary care physician before taking MSM to ensure their safety and avoid any potential complications. Taking this precaution is vital to protect one's health and prevent any possible harm. It is always better to err on the side of caution to avoid any adverse outcomes.

Monitor for allergic reactions

Individuals taking Methylsulfonylmethane (MSM) should exercise caution as those who are sensitive to sulfur may develop an allergic reaction. Symptoms of an allergic reaction include hives, swelling, or difficulty breathing and require immediate medical attention.

MSM may also interact with certain medications such as blood thinners and anti-inflammatory drugs. It is best to consult with a healthcare provider before taking MSM to ensure it is safe for individual use.

Store properly

To maximize the benefits of Methylsulfonylmethane (MSM) supplements, it is crucial to handle and store them properly. MSM should be kept in a dry and cool place away from direct sunlight, as heat and moisture can diminish its effectiveness. Additionally, it is essential to check the seal before using the product.

If the seal is absent or appears to be tampered with, it is best not to use the MSM supplement as it could be contaminated and unsafe for consumption. By taking these simple safety precautions and considerations, individuals can ensure that they are getting the most out of their MSM supplements while avoiding potential health risks.

By following these safety precautions and considerations, you can ensure that your MSM supplementation is safe and effective. Always consult with a healthcare provider before taking any new supplement or medication to avoid potential side effects or interactions.

Speak with them if you experience any adverse effects after starting MSM supplementation. They can help you find the right dose for your individual needs and provide guidance on how to safely use MSM for the best results.

Who Can Take Methylsulfonylmethane (MSM)

MSM is generally considered safe for most adults when taken as directed. However, as with any supplement, certain groups may need to exercise caution or talk to their doctor before taking MSM. Here are some guidelines regarding who can take MSM:

Healthy Adults

Because it helps reduce inflammation, boost immunological function, and maintain healthy skin, hair, and nails, methylsulfonylmethane (MSM) is an all-natural and risk-free method for promoting overall health and wellness. Because it has been found to potentially enhance energy levels and improve exercise performance, it is an excellent addition to a healthy lifestyle and should be considered an essential component.

Athletes and fitness enthusiasts

Because it helps prevent muscular damage, soreness, and joint pain caused by vigorous activity, MSM can be a valuable supplement for athletes and fitness lovers. MSM can be found at almost any health food store. It is also believed to promote joint flexibility and mobility, which in turn enables individuals to perform better during workouts and recover from them more rapidly.

People with arthritis

People who suffer from inflammatory joint disorders such as osteoarthritis and rheumatoid arthritis may find relief from their joint pain, swelling, and stiffness with the use of MSM. Arthritis sufferers may see an improvement in their quality of life as a result of the medication's ability to reduce joint inflammation and support healthy joint function.

People with skin conditions

Due to the anti-inflammatory and antioxidant characteristics that MSM possesses, it has been applied directly to the skin in order to treat a variety of skin diseases. As a result of its potential to alleviate symptoms of acne, rosacea, and eczema and to improve the appearance of healthy, youthful skin, it is used as a component in a wide variety of skincare products.

People with digestive issues

MSM has the potential to enhance digestive function and alleviate symptoms of digestive illnesses such as irritable bowel syndrome and leaky gut syndrome. It does this by protecting the lining of the digestive tract and lowering inflammation there, which in turn may improve symptoms and the health of the digestive tract as a whole.

Overall, while MSM is generally considered safe for most adults, it is important to approach it with caution and talk to your doctor before taking it if you have any underlying health conditions or are taking medication. By following dosage instructions carefully and choosing a high-quality supplement from a reputable manufacturer, you can safely and effectively enjoy the potential benefits of MSM.

Food Sources of Methylsulfonylmethane (MSM)

Methylsulfonylmethane (MSM) is naturally found in certain foods, so it's possible to get some of your MSM from dietary sources. Here are some food sources of MSM:

Fruits and vegetables

Broccoli, Brussels sprouts, kale, spinach, tomatoes, and apples are packed with vital nutrients, including MSM in small amounts. MSM is a sulfur-containing compound that plays a crucial role in human health. These foods are an excellent source of MSM that can enhance joint function, reduce inflammation, and promote healthy skin and hair.

Meats and seafood

Poultry, beef, and fish are excellent sources of MSM, a compound known for its beneficial effects on joint health. Among fish, salmon, sardines, and anchovies are particularly high in MSM, as well as omega-3 fatty acids, which are important for heart and brain health. These types of fish are also low in mercury and other contaminants, making them a safe and healthy choice for those looking to boost their MSM intake.

Nuts and seeds

Almonds, walnuts, and sesame seeds are excellent sources of Methylsulfonylmethane (MSM). These nutrient-rich foods not only contain MSM, but also provide healthy fats, protein, and fiber. Consuming these nuts and seeds regularly can significantly boost one's MSM intake, offering numerous health benefits.

Legumes

Lentils, chickpeas, and black beans are the richest sources of Methylsulfonylmethane (MSM), providing numerous health benefits. Moreover, they are packed with plant-based protein, fiber, iron, zinc, and folate, making them ideal additions to any healthy diet. Consuming a diet rich in these legumes may help alleviate inflammation, reduce oxidative stress, enhance joint health, and promote optimal wellness.

Whole grains

Whole grains like brown rice, quinoa, and oats contain small amounts of MSM. They are also a good source of fiber, complex carbohydrates, and other important nutrients.

It's worth noting that the amount of MSM found naturally in these foods is relatively low compared to the dosage typically used in supplements. So while incorporating these foods into your diet can be a good way to get some additional MSM, it may not provide the same level of benefits as taking an MSM supplement.

How diet can play a role in getting enough Methylsulfonylmethane (MSM)

Diet can play a role in getting enough MSM, although it may not provide the same level of benefits as taking an MSM supplement. MSM is found in small amounts in a variety of foods, including fruits, vegetables, grains, and animal products. Here are a few ways to incorporate MSM-rich foods into your diet:

1. *Eat a variety of fruits and vegetables:* Incorporating a wide range of fruits and vegetables into your diet can help increase your intake of MSM. Some of the best sources of MSM include broccoli, Brussels sprouts, kale, spinach, tomatoes, and apples. These foods are also rich in other important vitamins, minerals, and antioxidants that support overall health.
2. *Choose lean meats and seafood:* Lean cuts of meat like chicken and turkey, as well as fish like salmon and sardines, are good sources of MSM. Choosing lean protein sources can help reduce your intake of unhealthy fats while also increasing your MSM intake. Additionally, fish like salmon and sardines also contain

omega-3 fatty acids which have numerous health benefits.
3. ***Snack on nuts and seeds:*** Nuts and seeds like almonds, walnuts, and sesame seeds are another great source of MSM. These foods can be easily incorporated into your diet by snacking on them throughout the day or adding them to salads, oatmeal, or yogurt.
4. ***Incorporate legumes into your diet:*** Legumes like lentils, chickpeas, and black beans are high in both fiber and protein, making them an excellent addition to any diet. They are also a good source of MSM and can be added to soups, stews, and salads.
5. ***Choose whole grains:*** Whole grains like brown rice, quinoa, and oats contain small amounts of MSM but are also rich in other important nutrients like fiber, vitamins, and minerals. Switching to whole-grain versions of bread, pasta, and cereal can help boost your overall intake of MSM and other essential nutrients.

While diet alone may not provide the same level of benefits as taking an MSM supplement, incorporating these MSM-rich foods into your diet can help ensure that you're getting some MSM naturally. It's important to consult with a healthcare professional before starting any new supplement regimen, especially if you have any underlying health conditions or are taking medications.

Conclusion

Congratulations! You've made it to the end of our in-depth look into methylsulfonylmethane, also known as MSM. You've undoubtedly reached the point where you're asking how come you haven't heard about this fantastic compound earlier. You need not be concerned about missing out on any information on MSM because we are here to fill you in.

MSM offers a wide range of benefits, some of which include lowering joint pain and inflammation, improving skin health, and enhancing exercise performance. Because of this, you should give some thought to using MSM as one of your daily supplements. And let's be honest: who doesn't want to improve how they feel, make their movements smoother, and progress to the next level in their workouts?

But before you start including MSM in your arsenal of supplements, it is vital to keep in mind that research into the full effects of this natural component is still underway. This is something you should keep in mind before beginning to use MSM. Even though there is a wealth of encouraging information available, it is always best practice to approach with caution and seek the advice of a qualified medical practitioner prior to beginning any new supplement routine.

After consulting with your primary care physician and receiving confirmation that it is okay for you to consume MSM, the next step is to search for an MSM supplement of superior quality that is tailored to your specific requirements. You should look for companies that employ MSM that are of pure and high quality, and you should follow the dosage directions that are listed on the product's label.

Also, keep in mind that having more does not necessarily make something better. Maintain the dosages that are prescribed for you, and pay special attention to any changes in your health or symptoms.

But don't worry if taking dietary supplements isn't your thing! MSM can also be found in its naturally occurring state in a wide variety of foods, including fruits, vegetables, grains, and products derived from animals. You may assist ensure that you are getting some MSM naturally by including these foods that are rich in MSM in your diet; but, the advantages that you receive from doing so may not be on par with those that you receive from taking an MSM supplement.

What exactly are you looking forward to? MSM has something beneficial to offer everyone, whether you're an athlete trying to boost your performance or just someone battling with joint pain and inflammation. MSM has something for everyone. Give it a shot, and observe how it affects the state of your health and wellness as a whole.

And who can say for sure? It's possible that the missing piece of the puzzle will turn out to be MSM, so keep an open mind. Imagine being able to run that additional mile, feeling comfortable while you go about your daily activities, or sleeping better at night. All of these things are possible. It's that MSM is the answer you've been looking for all along.

In conclusion, MSM is an encouraging naturally occurring molecule that has a great deal to offer in terms of enhancing one's overall health and sense of well-being. Even though the research is not yet complete, the first findings have produced a lot of excitement. Always check with your doctor before beginning a new supplement routine, and make sure to pick products that have a good reputation and use only pure MSM in their formulations. Therefore, there is no reason to hold back; give MSM a shot, and be ready to take your overall health and fitness to the next level!

FAQ

What exactly is MSM?

MSM, which stands for methylsulfonylmethane, is a naturally occurring molecule that may be found in trace levels in a variety of foods. It is also consumed as a dietary supplement in the hope that it will enhance skin health, promote joint health, and reduce inflammation.

What are some of the possible advantages of using MSM?

MSM is a nutritional supplement that is often used to enhance joint health, reduce inflammation, and improve skin health. MSM also has antimicrobial properties. It's also possible that it has antioxidant effects and helps the immune system work better.

How do I take MSM?

MSM can be obtained in a number of different formulations, such as capsules, pills, powders, and topical lotions. It is normally used orally, and the dosage that is advised will vary depending on the particular product that is being used. Never deviate from the dose instructions provided on the product label or from what your healthcare provider tells you to take.

Is the MSM safe to consume?

When used in the recommended dosage, MSM is not thought to pose any health risks. On the other hand, it has the potential to induce adverse effects in some individuals, including problems with the digestive system, headaches, and weariness.

Before beginning to take MSM, it is essential to discuss the supplement with a qualified medical professional, particularly if you are currently managing any preexisting medical conditions or are taking any drugs.

Is it possible to apply MSM topically?

MSM is indeed formulated into topical creams, which can be used to directly apply the compound to the skin. It is frequently used in skin care products in the hope that it will improve the health of the skin and reduce inflammation.

Does MSM have the potential to interact with other medications?

There is a possibility that MSM will interact negatively with a number of treatments, including chemotherapeutic drugs and immunosuppressants. If you are already on medicine, it is critical that you have a conversation with your healthcare provider before beginning to use MSM.

Where exactly can I find MSM?

MSM supplements are able to be purchased from a variety of sources, including health food stores, online sellers, and some pharmacies. Additionally, it can be found in various fruits and vegetables, lean meats, nuts, seeds, and legumes, albeit in much lower concentrations than in other foods.

References and Helpful Links

Berry, J. (2023, May 24). Health benefits and possible side effects of MSM (methylsulfonylmethane).
https://www.medicalnewstoday.com/articles/324544

Stuart, A. (2013, February 6). MSM (Methylsulfonylmethane).

Barmaki, S., Bohlooli, S., Khoshkhahesh, F., & Nakhostin-Roohi, B. (2012). Effect of methylsulfonylmethane supplementation on exercise Induced muscle damage and total antioxidant. . . ResearchGate.
https://www.researchgate.net/publication/224824181_Effect_of_methylsulfonylmethane_supplementation_on_exercise_Induced_muscle_damage_and_total_antioxidant_capacity

Northrop, A. (2023, May 17). MSM Supplements: Benefits And Risks (Methylsulfonylmethane). Forbes Health.
https://www.forbes.com/health/body/msm-supplements/#:~:text=May%20Help%20Treat%20Seasonal%20Allergies,of%20MSM%20for%2030%20days.

Withee, E. D., Tippens, K. M., Dehen, R., Tibbitts, D., Hanes, D., & Zwickey, H. (2017b). Effects of Methylsulfonylmethane (MSM) on exercise-induced oxidative stress, muscle damage, and pain following a half-marathon: a double-blind, randomized, placebo-controlled trial. Journal of the International Society of Sports Nutrition, 14(1). https://doi.org/10.1186/s12970-017-0181-z

Rd, J. K. M. (2023, February 1). 8 Science-Backed Benefits of MSM Supplements. Healthline. https://www.healthline.com/nutrition/msm-supplements#:~:text=MSM%20may%20help%20reduce%20pain,helping%20you%20recover%20more%20quickly.

www.ingramcontent.com/pod-product-compliance
Lightning Source LLC
LaVergne TN
LVHW051925060526
838201LV00062B/4685